HYDI
GARDEN SECRET

THE SECRET TO HAVING YOUR FRUITS AND VEGETABLES IN ALL SEASONS WITH THE HYDROPONIC GARDEN. HOW TO GROW PERFECT PLANTS ALL YEAR ROUND

©Copyright 2020 Susanne Parker - All rights reserved.

The content contained within this book may not be reproduced, duplicated or transmitted without direct written permission from the **author** or the publisher.

Under no circumstances will any blame or legal responsibility be held against the publisher, or author, for any damages, reparation, or monetary loss due to the information contained within this book. Either directly or indirectly.

Legal Notice:

This book is copyright protected. This book is only for personal use. You cannot amend, distribute, sell, use, quote or paraphrase any part, or the content within this book, without the consent of the author or publisher.

Disclaimer Notice:

Please note the information contained within this document is for educational and entertainment purposes only. All effort has been executed to present accurate, up to date, and reliable, complete information. No warranties of any kind are declared or implied. Readers acknowledge that the author is not engaging in the rendering of legal, financial, medical or professional advice. The content within this book has been derived from various sources. Please consult a licensed professional before attempting any techniques outlined in this book.

By reading this document, the reader agrees that under no circumstances is the author responsible for any losses, direct or indirect, which are incurred as a result of the use of information contained within this document, including, but not limited to, — errors, omissions, or inaccuracies.

Table of Contents

Introduction 5

Chapter 1: Hydroponic Cultivation 10

Chapter 2: History of Hydroponic 14

Chapter 3: Advantages and Disadvantages of Hydroponic 20

Chapter 4: Different Types of Hydroponic Gardens .. 29

    Wicking systems 30

    Deep-water culture (DWC) systems 32

    Nutrient film technique (NFT) systems 36

    Ebb and flow / flood and drain systems 38

    Aeroponics systems 40

    Drip systems 41

Chapter 5: How to Build your Hydroponic System 43

    Essentiality of hydroponic farming 48

Chapter 6: Operating Cycle 53

Chapter 7: The Best Plants for Hydroponic Gardening 59

Chapter 8: Maintenance 71

    Cleanliness 71

Nutrient Solution 73

Watering 74

Reservoir Temperature 75

Humidity 75

Inspect the Equipment 76

Look at Your Plants 81

Change One Thing at a Time 83

Chapter 9: The Myths and Errors to Avoid 85

Chapter 10: Hydroponics vs. Soil Gardening 95

Chapter 11: Making Money from Your Greenhouse 106

Chapter 12: Tips, Tricks, and Hacks to Always Grow Healthy Plants in Your Garden 116

Other tips and tricks to know when running a hydroponic system: 122

Final Words 127

Introduction

It is an understatement to say that without water, human existence is equated to nothing. That is, water is life. There would be no hydroponics to practice or creating a society of it. Water is an essential part of all living cells. This induces turgor pressure on cell walls of plants to prevent the leaves from wilting. And it holds nutrients and energy reserves all over the plant in the form of dissolved salts and sugars. This is about water, focusing on how it is being distributed, how to preserve its consistency, and how to supplement it with plant life's essential nutrients. Fire and water work together in nature so as to recharge the soil with nutrients. Woods turns to ash as trees burn in the forest. Wood ash is high in Potassium, one of the essential nutrients of the plant kingdom. Lifeless leaves and fallen branches are helped on their path to decline when the rains come. This cycle is intensified by animals and insects by eating plant materials and excreting organic waste that filters down into the soil below. The organic matter in the soil is bio-decomposed into the basic nutrient salts on which the plants feed. The dropping rains continue to remove these salts once again, making them available for plants to consume from their roots. Everything in nature should be in perfect harmony if a plant is to be provided a well-balanced or adequately balanced diet. Forests must burn, cattle must feed, rains must fall, the wood must rot, and there must be bacteria in the soil and ready to go to work.

You will never ever see these ideal conditions happening regularly. Besides, the rainforests of the world might be the only remaining examples of near-perfect botanical conditions.

Now that we grasp the natural growing process better, we can see that hydroponics is all about enriching water with the very same nutritional salts found in nature. It's about creating and maintaining a perfectly balanced "nutrient solution" for your plants. Many hydroponic systems have a closed system that stores the nutrient solution. It helps protect it from evaporation and pollution into our atmosphere, just as the wastewater from untreated fertilized soil does. This conservative approach to water management makes hydroponics the tool of choice in drought-stricken areas around the world, and as a result, it is quickly becoming recognized as "Earth Friendly Farming." Since you will be learning the art and science of "climate farming," it is a good idea to know what your local water contains. Contact your local water company and request their analysis of water quality. If your water comes from a well, you'll most likely have to take it out to your own laboratory for study. The relative "hardness" or "softness" is the most important factor influencing water quality. Hard water means that there is a lot of dissolved mineral content, mostly calcium carbonate, and is often seen as a scale on hot water pipes. Soft water in dissolved solids is usually very pure, or weak. Distilled (or deionized) water, or water going through a tank for reverse osmosis, is all called liquid. Most of the marketable hydroponic products are made for soft water. If you have hard water, though, there are some nutrient items that are also designed for hard water.

Is Hydroponics worth the while?

Gardeners enjoy hydroponics because it's possible to grow almost anything, and there's little or no backbreaking work: no tilling, raking or hoeing. There are no pulling of weeds and no spraying of toxic pesticides. Few moles or cutworms consume the roots, and most insects leave their plants clean and healthy alone.

Hydroponics is suitable for the homeowner or tenant hobbyists who have no time or space for full-time gardening of the land. In late spring and summer, you can place your portable hydroponic unit outside on a porch or balcony where natural sunlight helps to produce tremendous yields from lettuce, to cucumbers, to zinnias. The unit can be moved anywhere inside the home in winter, even into the basement, where your plants will thrive and continue to be produced under artificial light.

Plants love to grow through hydroponics because their roots don't have to pass through thick, chunky soil to fight for nutrients. Alternatively, one hydroponic system equally distributes nutrients to each vine. Plants also need oxygen to breathe, and a porous expanding aggregate, unlike dirt, allows air to circulate around them freely. And everything is growing fast and beautifully.

Hydroponic plants grow quicker, mature earlier, and give up the yield of soil-grown plants by up to ten times. This washed and pampered plants produce high nutritional value fruits and vegetables, with outstanding flavor. Many of them, particularly hydroponic tomatoes and cucumbers, are sold at far higher prices than ordinary vegetables in the gourmet part of supermarkets. The point here is that the same vegetables can be grown for considerably less money than the pulpy supermarket variety costs to buy.

Chapter 1: Hydroponic Cultivation

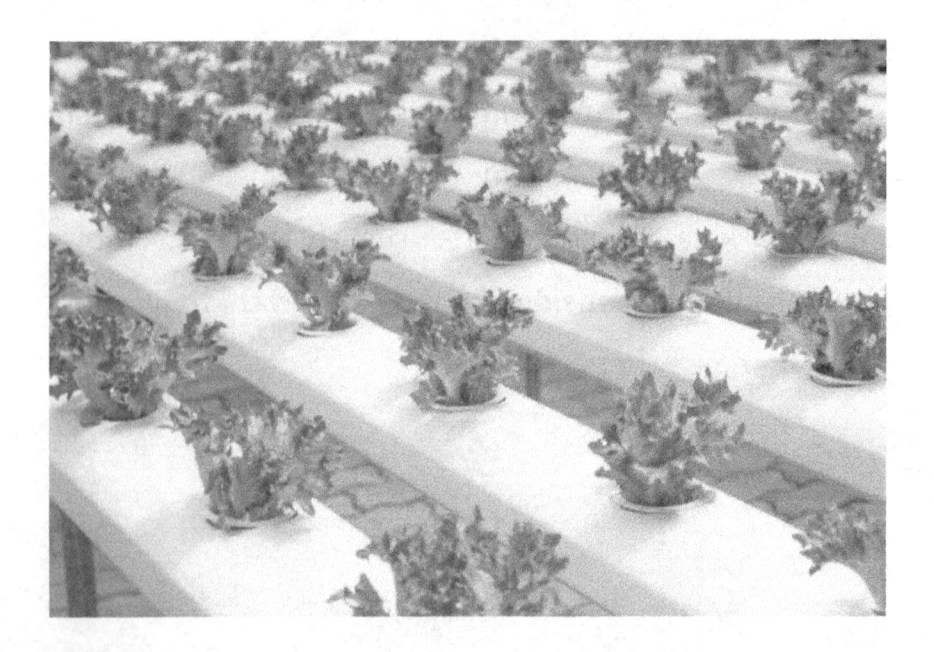

Hydroponics is a generic term that embraces different cultivation techniques that have as a standard feature the use of water and nutrients to feed plants that are grown "out of the soil" or without using the land.

There are two main methods of hydroponic cultivation; the first foresees the use of "inert" materials or supports whose purpose is only to support the root system of the plant, the other is the direct immersion of the roots in the nutrient solution.

The advantages of hydroponic without soil cultivation - compared to traditional cultivation techniques - lie above all in the possibility of starting one or more hydroponic crops even in less hospitable environments and in conditions not suitable for the birth and growth of plants. For example, it is indicated in all those places characterized by a high drought or where temperatures are particularly rigid or in areas where the soil under excessively sandy, rocky, or arid.

Amount of water to be provided for irrigation

Another essential aspect of hydroponic cultivation fundamental for fans and professionals of hydroponic gardening is the quantity of water to be provided for irrigation: in traditional crops on the land, the amount of water necessary to be able to cultivate and make the plants fruit is clearly higher compared to that required by vegetables grown in hydroponics. In fact, it is calculated that the ratio is 10 (for traditional crops) to 1 (for hydroponic crops).

Hydroponic culture

The saving of water is reflected both in the economic aspect and on the environmental issue.

In short, hydroponic cultivation - also known as hydroponic culture precisely because it affects different economic, social, and even cultural areas - has a decidedly limited ecological footprint compared to traditional cultivation techniques.

Use of fertilizers, herbicides, and pesticides

Another critical factor is the use of fertilizers, herbicides, and pesticides used and the relative quantities foreseen in the two types of crops: the volumes of fertilizers used are somewhat limited and always well targeted. Furthermore, there is no dispersion of the soil. Herbicides are not used, because they are not necessary, while pesticides are used in small quantities.

Organic Hydroponic cultivation

For those who want to grow organically, it is possible to use organic fertilizers that allow you to have a hydroponic organic culture, respecting health, and the environment.

Why choose a Hydroponic cultivation method?

In a Hydroponic system, plants grow out of the ground, in a fully regulated crop context and free from pests and diseases from the soil.

By controlling environmental parameters, such as light, nutrients, temperature, pH, and conductivity, results are obtained much higher than traditional crops, without having to use pesticides that often produce harmful effects on the culture itself.

The hydroponic cultivation technique maximizes the yield in terms of quality, quantity, and speed. For this reason, hydroponic crops are becoming increasingly popular and appreciated not only by professionals and large distribution chains (we point out that most of the tomatoes on sale today in supermarkets come from hydroponics) both from small direct growers and - for pleasure or work - they decide to try their hand at crops of this type.

Chapter 2: History of Hydroponic

Hydroponics is by no means a new addition to humanity. It dates back several thousand years, with the **Hanging Gardens** of Babylon producing the first known cases in the world in history. These gardens were designed to hang over the Euphrates River in Babylonia. They were able to bring up water for the plants in this setting with a pulley system that would allow for it to flow up the system. The water would then be pulled and dumped onto the steps of the garden to pour down and provide the plants with the water that they would need. Ultimately, people and plants have a very dependent nature to each other, and that leads to people naturally trying to figure out how best to cultivate their own for consumption.

In the city of Tenochtitlan, an ancient Aztec city in Mexico in the 10th century, people made use of floating farms that were suspended atop water to allow for the plants to grow. This allowed for them not to have to transfer the water that they had to shore—rather, and they could grow the plants atop the water and save that middle step.

Even more modernly, Marco Polo, the late 13th-century explorer, found that there were other floating gardens during travels in China.

Ultimately, however, it was not until the 1600s that you started to see scientific experiments surrounding the process of how plants grow, what they need, and how to facilitate that growth. It began with Belgian Jan Van Helmont, experimenting with plant growth and positing that ultimately, plants grow because they can absorb substances from water. However, this failed to acknowledge the fact that plants have two other common needs as well—they need carbon dioxide and oxygen, commonly absorbed through the air.

In 1699, just before the turn of the century, John Woodward began to experiment as well. He wanted to know how best to grow plants in water cultures, and he eventually determined that the water with the most soil in it allowed for the greatest development of plants in the first place. They thrived with the soil mixed in, likely because ultimately, those plants are the ones that will also include the minerals that soil brings with them. He assumed that the water absorbed the substances from the soil, and that then allowed the plants to grow further.

Similar studies continued throughout the years, and ultimately, in 1804, De Saussure, a scientist, assumed that plants were built up of the chemical elements that they absorbed from three places—the water, the soil, and the air. They seemed to be dependent upon all three to grow and develop properly. This was eventually verified in 1851 by a French chemist by the name of Boussignault. He ran an experiment in which he attempted to grow plants with several different insoluble media, such as sand, quartz, and charcoal. He made use of the water to hold the plants, the media, and then chemical nutrients. This was sort of the precursor to what we know as being the hydroponics process we know and love today. He discovered the need for water is due to the attainment of hydrogen from it.

Shortly after, in 1860, two German botanists discovered the proper formula that would allow for the dissolving of them into water that would allow for the growth of plants. Julius von Sachs and Wilhelm Knop created this process and formula and created the art of mariculture, which is known now as water culture. This allowed for the use of submerging the plants' roots entirely into a solution that was made to contain several minerals—the macronutrients that they need to grow.

This system was commonly used in experiments but did not get mainstream attention for quite some time. It was not until the mainstreaming of greenhouses that saw the increase in the application of mariculture practice in 1925. Here, people began to take notice of the fact that soil culture can be difficult and unsustainable. Because soil culture would involve problems in soil structure while also threatening the unpredictability of nature, causing problems, the attention turned to large-scale water cultivation to try to eliminate it.

However, it was not until the early 1930s that W.F. Gericke, a professor at the University of California at Berkeley, began to experiment with the processes for mariculture for crop production. He saw this as something that could happen. Initially, He tried to coin the term aquaculture at first—but ultimately settled down on the name of hydroponics after the suggestion from a coworker. Thus, hydroponics as a practice was born, and he repeatedly proved that it was one that could be used with relative reliability. While his coworkers and colleagues were skeptical, it took the use of the hydroponic system to grow a 25-foot-tall tomato plant to make other people see that this could be useful.

Of course, the university was still dubious at best, and ultimately, he was found to have been cultivating the plants all along after demanding that other students investigate whether this was a possibility or not. In 1938, the method was repeated, and hydroponics were found to be legitimate. However, they also deemed that the process of hydroponics did not change the fact that the plants produced similar quality fruit, completely missing and disregarding the fact that ultimately. Hydroponics also offers plenty of other benefits that could be greatly useful to the average person.

In the 1940s, however, there was the use made to hydroponically cultivate an entire island that was soilless in the Pacific Ocean. The island was commonly used as a refueling stop for Pan American Airlines. Still, due to the lack of soil, ti was incredibly difficult and expensive ever to get fresh vegetables or fruits present. However, with the use of hydroponics, they were able to cultivate the area making use of these methods, allowing for fresh vegetables to be provided after all.

This continued after WWII in Japan—entirely hydroponic gardens began to pop up all around the world.

Nowadays, using hydroponic farming is becoming much more popular. It provides higher growth rates, saves space, and allows for efficiency and a lack of loss, making it widely appreciated and desired. The vast majority of farms that make the use of greenhouses will make use of these sorts of methods, and so far, they are becoming incredibly commonplace.

Chapter 3: Advantages and Disadvantages of Hydroponic

Improved genetic health

Plants in a hydroponic system are not only provided with nutrition that has a near to perfect composition, but they're also safeguarded from many potential pests that they could otherwise come into contact with when growing in soil. This allows the plants to reach a higher level of genetic health. As the saying goes, 'you are what you eat.'

High-scale production

Although hydroponics can be used to create your variety of plants at home, an often-surprising fact is that the hydroponic process is responsible for providing food to millions. The science has now been improved to a level at which more fruit, vegetables, and herbs can be produced at a higher quality than ever before! Yields from growing hydroponically are at least 20% greater than with growing with soil.

Affordable

Hydroponics will allow you to say goodbye to the often-costly ordeals of obtaining prepared soils and plant protection products. On top of this, most of the standard gardening tools (e.g. trowels, shovels, forks) are not needed.

Less-time, more produce

The process of planting becomes a breeze because you will no longer have to spend time preparing soil between planting. On top of this, your plants will be able to mature faster, generating you an abundance of beautiful produce.

Vegetables, fruits, and flowers grow healthier

With hydroponics, plants get the right kinds of nutrient in the right amounts at the right time, which means that they contain the correct nutrient values in the produce. Studies show that there is 50% more nutritive content in crops grown in hydroponic gardens in contrast to traditional ones.

Faster, better results are achieved

Since nutrients are introduced and adjusted in the water, the plants feed directly and do not expend much energy tracing and extracting needed supply of nutrients. They grow faster, bigger, and in superior quality. In this sterile, controlled environment, you will get double the yield from your crops.

Hydroponic gardens are easy to maintain

You can have a soil-less garden indoor or outdoor. You require less labor in the set-up and upkeep of a hydroponic garden. You don't need to test your soil or set up a plot. You can also use commercially available pH-balanced nutrient solutions.

You can grow and enjoy your crops

A lot of people worry about the chemical content in their food because of inorganic fertilizers, insecticides, and other plant sprays. Growing your vegetables and fruits at home can give you peace of mind that what you are eating is fresh and free from chemicals.

In a hydroponic garden, it is easy to harvest vegetables, fruits, and flowers. Moreover, you save more money.

You can grow plants anywhere

You only need a growing medium, water system, nutrient solution, and a light source, and you're good to go. Remember that plants will grow as long as their needs are met.

You save space

Unlike in soil gardens, you cannot have plants grow too close together or they will fight each other for nutrients. In a hydroponic garden, you can place plants with small roots together, and they will grow just as big and healthy as a traditional garden.

You help protect the environment

Traditional gardening leads to the degradation of soils as high amounts of potassium, phosphorus, and calcium are introduced to it through fertilizers. Hydroponics is a good way to reduce the amount of arable land.

Also, you need far less water for a hydroponic garden than you would in a soil-based one which contributes to conserving our Earth's water.

Hydroponic gardening is fun and relaxing

Hydroponic gardening is advantageous not only to commercial farmers but to home gardeners and those who are looking for hobbies, as well. Soil-less gardening is a fun, innovative, and great way to relax or spend time with your family. Additionally, there is much less physical labor involved in hydroponic gardening as compared to conventional gardening. It is a great stress reliever, as well. What can be more relaxing and rewarding than seeing the fruits of your labor literally, right in your own home?

There is little chance of environmental degradation

Fertilizers are not required in hydroponic farming. Additionally, you don't need to worry about changing seasons and weather conditions. Often, bad weather leads to the destruction of prized plants, flowers, and crops that you've worked so hard to cultivate, but with a hydroponic system you can avoid these natural disasters.

There is very little wastage of resources in hydroponic farming

Waste products are reduced because dirt and soil are not utilized. Water is easily disposed of in a clean and proper way. This reduces the possibility of over or under-watering. The supply of nutrient water is regulated; therefore, you will not have to double-check if the water is enough or not

The money you invest in preparing a garden and maintaining it is returned through produce which you can eat or sell for profit.

Safer and less need for the use of pesticides and chemicals

With hydroponic gardening, you also eliminate the possibility of pest infestation, therefore also removing the use of pesticides. This leads to a much healthier garden and products.

Improved home environment

Hydroponic gardens are some of the most beautiful gardens to have in your home. You can drastically improve the look of your environment through hydroponic gardening. Just as the site of an aquarium in your house is breathtaking, so it is the site of plants in your home.

The relieved strain on your budget

Food is expensive, even more so are fresh fruits and vegetables. You can make a great cut in your household budget by simply utilizing your free space by having a hydroponic garden.

Enriched skills

A Hydroponic garden is not just a garden, but a botanical laboratory of its own kind. You get to learn a lot about plants – how to take care of them, their basic requirements and how to maximize yields. You also learn how to utilize your farming skills as you get exercise and learn how to create a scenic, green landscape around your compound.

Cost of setup

Many traditional hydroponic setups can be quite expensive when you buy growing tents, lighting systems, and more. Although, prices are coming down due to LED lighting systems and other advances in technology. There are affordable hydroponic systems available, though you are limited in what can be grown in these.

Space requirements

Depending on the system you choose, it will need space indoors, perhaps in a garage or spare room. Some people will grow in their attic or basement, though if space is limited, look at the Ikea style growing systems which can be used on a kitchen countertop.

Learning curve

Growing in soil is relatively easy and, although there is a lot to learn, can be done without any expert knowledge. Hydroponic gardening does require some knowledge to choose the right type of lights, ensure they give out the right light spectrum at the right time, to monitor the pH levels and more. However, while this may sound complex to you, it is nowhere near as difficult as it sounds, and you will soon be comfortable with hydroponic growing.

Regular checking

You have to regularly check your hydroponic system, monitoring nutrient and pH levels. Initially, this may be quite difficult while you get used to it, but as you get used to hydroponic gardening, this will require less work. It can make vacations a little tricky, but most hydroponic systems will cope with being left alone for up to a week.

Water-based microorganisms

However, through proper hygiene and care the chances of this is minimal, particularly as you monitor the system regularly and can spot problems before they become serious.

Limited range of plants

Not all plants are suitable for growing in hydroponic systems, and depending on the method you are using, you may only be able to produce certain types of plants or only a single type of plant at a time.

Diseases spread rapidly

Because the plants are spaced closer together and can often be the same type, if any diseases should get into the system then they can spread very quickly. Should a disease be introduced, you will need to sterilize your entire system and start again. However, diseases are rare in hydroponic systems when proper hygiene is practiced, and new plants enter quarantine before introduction.

Chapter 4: Different Types of Hydroponic Gardens

Hydroponics is a collective concept for all growing methods in which a plant is rooted in a relatively thin layer by a large part of the organic substrate. The substrate itself is laid on a perforated base, which, in turn, is lowered into a trough (or tray) filled with a nutrient solution. Plant roots penetrate through the substrate layer and the openings of the base into the solution and thus satisfy the plant's need for food and water.

These are six main types of hydroponic systems.

Wicking systems

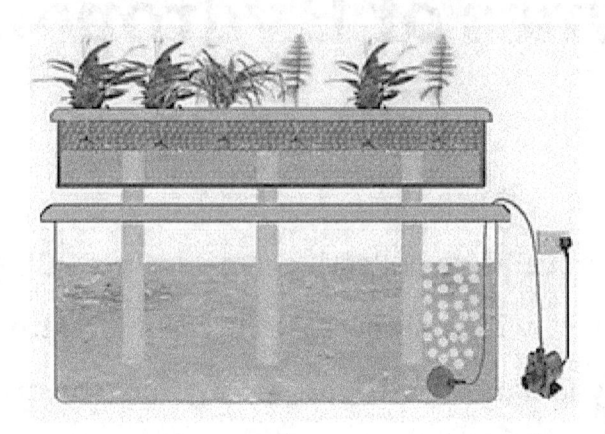

Record has it that the wick method is the simplest method in its formation and functions of all the other methods. Firstly, the wick system doesn't require electricity nor pumps because they don't possess any moving parts. The system is recommended because it's easy in that it only requires four components for its building of which daily household items can be used. People learning about hydroponics for the first time should definitely go for the wick system.

In the wick system, nutrient solutions are drawn up from the reservoir to the plants via a process called capillary action. The wick system is built in such a way that the growing container is placed a little distance just above the reservoir and then wicks are put in place so that they draw up the nutrient solution needed from the reservoir and then deliver into the growing medium that absorbs it and then supplies the plant roots with it. The capillary action is all the wick system needs to work.

However, the wick system as good and easy as it is does not work well with larger plants that need more water or heavy feeding plants that need nutrients supplied to their roots faster than how the wicks work. There must also be a regular flushing of excess nutrients from the growing media using plain fresh water to ensure there are no build-ups of mineral salts which are toxic.

Irrespective of the few downsides, the wick system is still highly recommended because of how uniquely simple it is. It allows for a great project for beginners just starting out with hydroponics. One of the topmost reasons people love and recommend this system is because of all the other systems, it is the most environmentally friendly one. In addition, the maintenance is easy; just regular checks to flush excess nutrients and to refill the nutrient solution in the reservoir. So, if you are about to grow small non-fruiting plants such as lettuce or herbs for personal or family consumption, wicks system is advisable.

Deep-water culture (DWC) systems

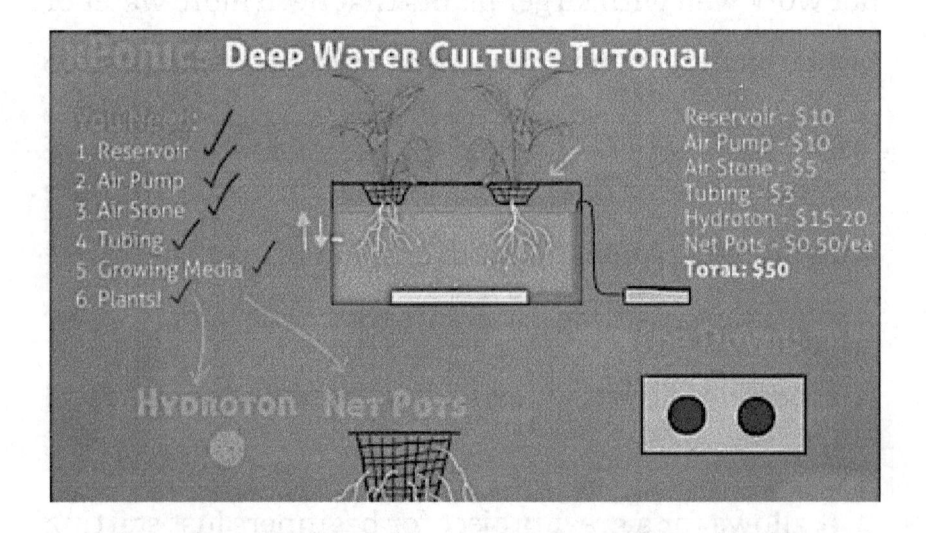

Another method that can be adopted in the hydroponics system is the deep-water culture. The system is also known as the direct water culture. This system is not like the aforementioned ones. In the deep-water culture system, the plant's roots are submersed into water. Moreover, in the deep-water culture, the roots are not just merely submersed in water and then the grower goes to sleep. The idea behind it is that there's a well oxygenated solution which is full of water and nutrients in which the roots are then dipped in. The truth is that in as much as people may fear taking chances because they feel the plant may die due to excess water; water when other essentials such as oxygen, nutrients, lights and appropriate temperature are provided for plant's root enable the plant to survive and flourish.

This system is a case of; more water, more firmness in nutrient solution, worry less about maintenance and monitoring. The necessity in this system is oxygen and this is provided either using an air pump or falling water which in turn brings about air bubbles that will rise from the dissolved water and the nutrient solution in the reservoir. While plants absorb sufficient oxygen, they are still able to take up adequate nutrients and water around it all their days. Hence, there is faster growth. The air pumps and the air stone must therefore work all day if not the plants get water-logged, run out of oxygen and then die.

The air stone is connected with the air pump through the airline and it's placed in the reservoir. Nutrients and water are then added and the plants that are put in net pots are placed above the nutrient solution in the reservoir. Once the roots touch the nutrient solution, there would be a growth outbreak. The water should be properly oxygenated so that the plant's root doesn't encounter any challenge and can actually remain in water for their whole life cycle. The reason the plants don't suffocate is because of the air and oxygen. This air and oxygen are present because of the air bubbles that rise through the nutrient solution and the dissolved oxygen in the water. Ensure there's as much air bubbles that make the water look as though it's boiling. When the air bubbles rise up to have a direct contact with the roots, then there's much effectiveness.

NUTRIENT FILM TECHNIQUE EXPLAINED

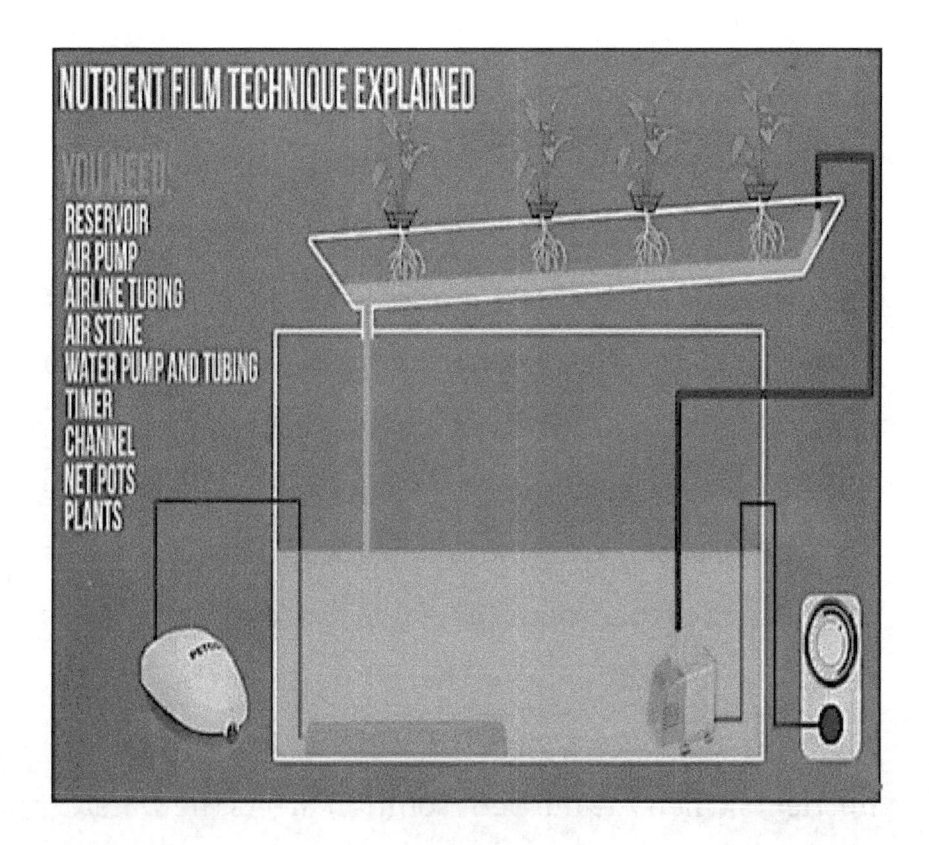

YOU NEED:
RESERVOIR
AIR PUMP
AIRLINE TUBING
AIR STONE
WATER PUMP AND TUBING
TIMER
CHANNEL
NET POTS
PLANTS

The most suitable plants to be grown in this method are plants that don't require flowering. Therefore, plants such as lettuce and other herbs are good for the system. Other fruits such as peppers, tomatoes and even squash that is a larger fruit can be grown using this method, however with increased effort.

Nutrient film technique (NFT) systems

The Nutrient film technique system is the next recommended hydroponics system for you. The system uses water pumps to deliver the nutrients to the plants. The NFT flows continuously. This system is an active one in that it needs moving parts to work and it provides the most effective conditions for plants to grow. The NFT has depthless nutrient solution that pours down through the tubing that then supplies the roots of the plants with nutrients when the nutrient solution meets the water.

The foliage sits on top of the plant roots that grow into a dense mat in the media. At times, there can be support given by a trellis system. The NFT delivers nutrients to the grow tray via a pump whilst a drained pipe is present to recycle the remnant water nutrient solution. This works when the grow tray is placed at a point (supported either by a rack or on a bench) to let the water nutrients flow down to the nutrient return pipe. The excess nutrient solution will then flow into another channel or tube and then a recirculation throughout the system takes place. In this system, the roots of the plants reach the bottom of the channel where they come in contact with the film of the nutrient solution and get nutrients from them. The thinness of the film nutrient solution allows the plants to be watered without being entirely soaked. The thinness also ensures the upper part of the roots have access to oxygen and are kept dry. The two main elements needed for the system are grow tray and reservoir.

The reservoir contains an air stone that is connected to an air pump that is placed outside the reservoir. This is done to oxygenate the water. There are two ends that connect the reservoir to the grow tray. There's the high end where the reservoir is connected to the grow tray through a nutrient pump and then at the low end, it's connected to the nutrient return pipe. The reservoir size depends on how much plants you want to grow. Also, since the NFT us a recirculating system, the reservoir is used to contain the nutrient solution. The water pumps used in this system do not have automatic timers that mean that it runs constantly. In order to avoid challenges that come with power failure or system failures, ensure you have a backup ready and also, check the pumps and fill the tubes regularly.

Ebb and flow / flood and drain systems

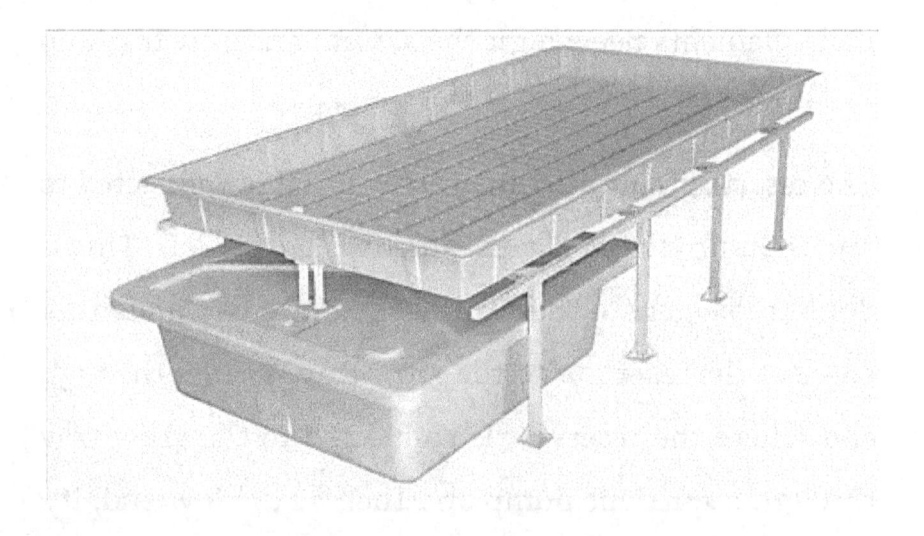

The next method of hydroponics is the ebb and flow. This system is also referred to as flood and drain and just as the name implies, it involves the frequent flooding and draining of the nutrient solutions. The flood operation involves the nutrient solutions flowing over the plant's roots while the drain involves the water being drained back to reservoir reservoirs. These basic actions uninterruptedly occur in this system. For the ebb and flow system to work, there are two major umbrella materials needed; which are the reservoir and the grow tray. There should be a nutrient solution reservoir which contains the nutrients and the water solution that the plants need, a submersible pump which is vital for pumping water into the grow tray. This is the center of the ebb and flow system, therefore, ensure that the pump you purchase has a strong flow rate that is capable of supplying the grow tray with water within short intervals. In addition, a timer is needed. It controls the amount of time for the watering process. This ensures the plants get the adequate nutrients they need.

Aeroponics systems

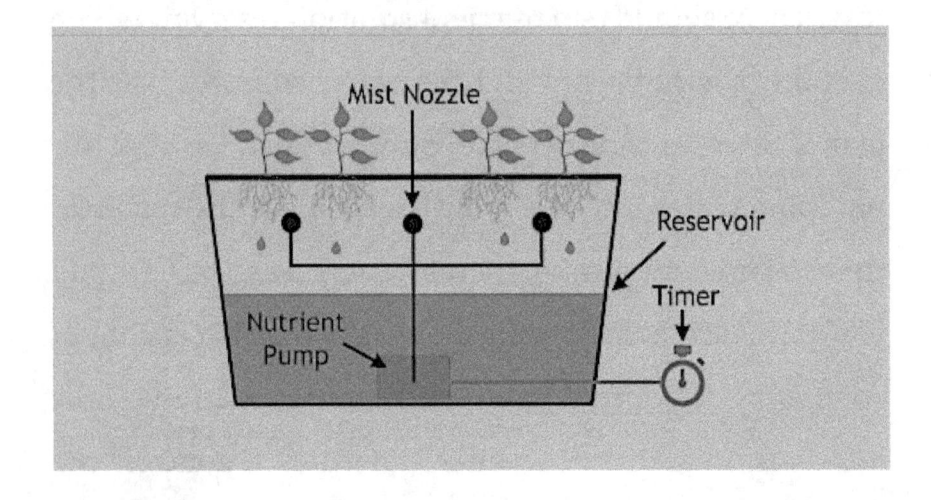

The next system of hydroponics we would be looking at is aeroponics. Aeroponics is a form of soilless cultivation which does not require the use of the soil as a medium for planting and harvesting. Aeroponics, which provides the advantages of increased water uptake by the plant, adequate aeration to the roots, and the reuse of nutrient solutions, has been mostly used in the cultivation of root crops especially in pharmaceutical industries. In practicing aeroponics, all that you need to be to ensure that the seeds are planted in foams which are then put in pots with perforated holes. The pots are exposed to light on one end and on the other end; they are exposed to a nutrient mist that are periodically supplied by pump system. Eventually, the roots of the plants are left to dangle in the air and are supplied water and nutrients by specific devices created for that purpose.

Drip systems

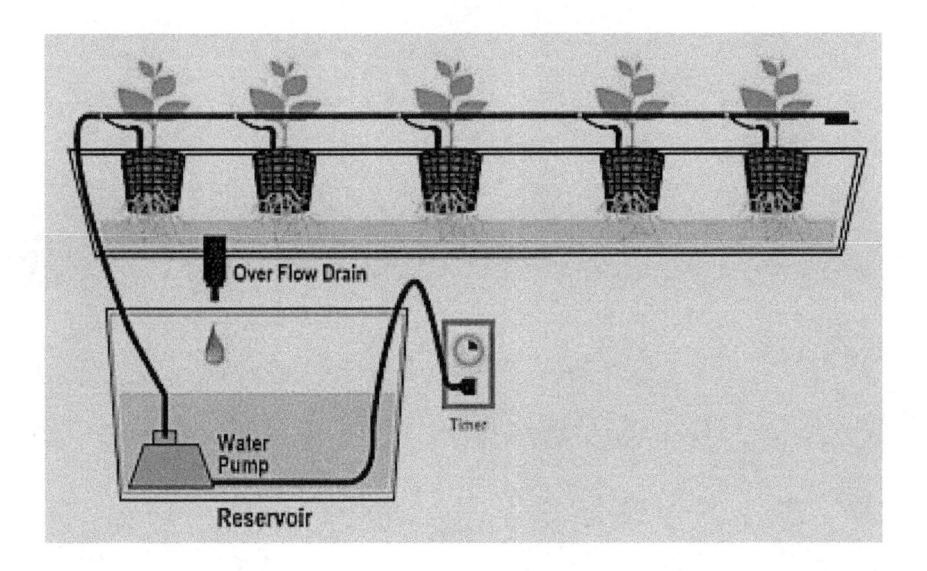

Another hydroponic system that can be adopted is the drip system. This system is an active one in that it makes use of pumps to supply the plants with the necessary nutrients and water regularly. With the drip system, you're allowed to control the amount of nutrients and water that are supplied to the plants. The supply is done via connecting feeder lines to deliver water for the plants. The system is most useful for large growing operations, the more reason why commercial growers prefer using it.

Chapter 5: How to Build your Hydroponic System

We know to build your hydroponic system is an arduous task to do. And especially if you have no experience and technical knowledge about the system, then it seems like an impossible task. But seriously there is nothing like impossible thing in building the hydroponic system because you only need to follow some simple steps and then you will get your hydroponic system without any error.

1) Determine the space/location

Indeed, one of the most essential and initial steps for building your hydroponic system. An excellent place or space where you want to establish your system is the path of attaining success. It doesn't matter whether you are developing your hydroponic system in your home or outside your home or in an open space area, the place should be leveled to maintain the right balance of the system.

If you are planning to locate the hydroponic system inside your home, then choose a dry place and a place which is far away from the electrical circuit. Though some of the systems run on electricity, you also need to remember that water will also be present in the system and any leakage can cause severe damage.

And if you want to locate your hydroponic system outside, then you have to must ensure the prevention of your network from outside elements like wind barrier, temperature and humidity level, protection from worms and other pests. And in the cold temperature, you need to bring your system inside your home to prevent the plants.

2) Assemble - Hydroponic System

Each hydroponic system has its specific design and structure. Some are highly equipped because of their commercial purpose, and some are like a wicking system which mainly made for house farming.

So, let's know about general hydroponic systems assemble process:

Your hydroponic system consists of with reservoir that is also known as container or tank, the tubes through which water and solution come, net pot or anything which holds the plants, water pump and stone which creates the bubbles, recycle the water and generate enough oxygen for the plants. Some other essential things like nutrients solutions. So, after getting all these things, then assemble them carefully.

3) Mixing of the nutrient solution in the tank Then fill up the tank with water. And after that add some needed amount of nutrients into the tub and turn on the pump so that water and nutrients solution will mix thoroughly.

4) Add Plants If you do not have any experience or time to grow seeds by yourself, then it would be best for you to purchase seeds from the market, and this is the most-simplest process of planting a hydroponic garden. But for more significant results, you need to choose a healthier plant root of your desire and then clean it thoroughly. It means to remove all the soil and dirt from the sources.

After that wash them gently and submerge the roots into the lukewarm water to cold water. Remember that too cold or hot water can damage the roots and give them initial shock that can cause unhealthier results. And then separate each root for removing the soil because any soil left can log the spray holes.

So, after cleaning the roots, pull the roots from the bottom of the cup of planting and add some stretched clay pebbles. These clays are hard and capable enough to hold the roots without any damage.

5) Tie the sources in the trellis

The next step involves the process of attaching the origins in the grille. For this, you can use strings and plant clips to tie the plant's roots to the trellis, because chains and clips can attain better support for the plant. And these are also helpful in maximizing the space. So, tie up the strings to the top of the roots through a grille, attach the clips at the bottom of the plant.

6) Turn the system on and monitor it

So, after completing all the steps, now turn on the water pump and monitor the system daily. We are saying because sometimes due to the evaporation or excessive heat, the system runs out of the water and in that particular situation the tank become dry and your pump can burn up too.

On the other hand, you also need to check the nutrients level and PH level in a regular interval of time.

7) Measure plant growth

Hydroponic farming or planting is the most significant way of getting quick and better results. Because the plant needs water and nutrients for overgrowing and through a hydroponic system, they consume it more rapidly. They grow faster, and that is why you need to monitor or measure plant growth every day.

8) Check the diseases and pests in the plant Disease and pests are one of the biggest obstacles in the process of hydroponics. Any bug or pests can destroy your hard work in a short period. Any foliar disease chewed leaves, and insect pest presence can damage your entire system.

So, it would be better for you to remove plant which is infected or sick immediately. Plants that grow hydroponically do not need to spend their energy to locate food because they automatically get the required food. That is why they spend their strengths to fight with the disease and with any infection.

Essentiality of hydroponic farming

1) Soilless growing

The story of hydroponic growing was started in 1940 when some researchers had introduced the phenomenon of the hydroponic system by growing vegetables without soil for the American troops. It was indeed a great and successful experiment in science. And now we all have been watching and gaining the benefits of landless growing or tank-based growing.

The most significant benefits of this method are that now we can grow plants and do farming where the soil is not appropriate for agriculture and gardening.

2) Space friendly

Yes, you can step up your hydroponic system wherever you want and can get some outstanding results of plantation or agriculture. If you wish to locate your order on the outside of your home or inside, it will give you the same results. Though you need to take care of some points like prevention from dirt and dust or faster wind because these can erupt the smooth progress of growing.

3) Control over climate conditions

The tradition farming or plantation mainly depends on the weather conditions and shows the growth according to the climate and seasons. That is why we get the vegetables and fruits available in the market according to the seasons.

But here the all process will be done on the tank or reservoir. It means you have total control over climate, seasons, weather conditions and air, temperature, and humidity. So, you can grow plants according to your need and also earn some high amount commercially.

4) Can save more water

Traditional farming or plantation requires more water consumption, and this is one of the biggest reasons why ground-level water degrading so much. A data says traditional farming method consumes around 80 percent of water in comparison to soilless growing. And if we talk about the hydroponic way, then it would be around 10 percent of water consumption. So, in this way, you can be able to save more water. Because there is only one way of water wasting in hydroponic and that is a leakage in the tank.

5) Maximum use of nutrients

Water and nutrients are the main elements which help the plant or roots to be healthy and multiply. But in the traditional method, the plant root takes more time and consumes fewer nutrients in comparison to soilless growing. The hydroponic system method shows the maximized use of nutrient solution and water for the plant's growth. By the hydroponic way, you can directly increase the water and nutrients into the roots of a plant, and by this, they will grow healthier and quicker.

6) PH control

Another great benefit of tank based growing in comparison of soil-based growing. Because here we can easily control the PH level of water and nutrients solutions more precisely and also can adjust them. And in this way, we can be able to ensure the number of nutrients consumed in the plant.

7) Greater growth rate

By giving the right atmosphere and climate condition, better nutrient, water supply, and light, you can quickly grow more plants than the traditional method. And hydroponics is the best way to provide a direct supply of mixed water and nutrient solution. And it is easily understandable that if you are providing all these things, then your growth rate will quickly become higher.

8) No Weed phenomenon

Yes, you heard it right. Because weeds develop in the soil and when you grow your plants hydroponically, then the aspect of weeds will be eradicated automatically. It means you can build your plants and do farming without any stress of weeds. Because, while doing the soil-based farming, we need to cut down the developed weeds from the soil to prevent the healthier growth of plants.

9) Prevention from diseases

Plant diseases such as fusarium, Pythium, and Rhizoctonia species destroys the healthiness of the plant and make them vulnerable. And pests such as groundhogs and gophers can also do severe damage in the plant growing. But if you are doing your farming through the tank method, then the chances of these things will be mitigated automatically.

10) Timesaving

In comparison to the traditional approach, you can save your significant amount of time through hydroponic farming. In the conventional method, you need to devote your time for watering, soil cultivation, and monitoring, but here you need to understand the equipment of tank-based farming. And the rest will be done by the system itself. By this, you can be able to save your time and your labor too.

11) Stress-free work Indeed, it is a stress-free way of doing farming of gardening. There is no need to do the soil cultivation or watering for the better soil condition. And you also need not devote your significant amount of time. However, you can do hydroponic farming as a hobby to make your life stress free.

Chapter 6: Operating Cycle

The growing process when you are using hydroponics is quite simple and does not differ too much from the traditional gardening growing process.

When you start your seeds, you will start them in a medium such as the oasis cubes. You will use whatever method you choose, placing them in the sun or under a grow light, but instead of simply watering them, you will give them the nutrient rich solution.

Once the seeds have sprouted and have taken root, you can transfer them to your hydroponics system, but you need to make sure that they are big enough for your specific system. You do not want to place your spouts in your system only to see them washed away or drowned so you should not rush the process of getting them into your hydroponics system.

Once the plants are in the hydroponics system, they will grow just as they would if you were growing them in a traditional garden.

The difference is that the plants are going to grow a lot faster than they would in a traditional garden and they are going to begin producing more fruit quicker than if they were in a traditional garden. Studies have shown that you can actually triple the amount of food that you are able to grow when you are using a hydroponics system versus traditional gardening.

When you think about how you are growing your plants, one of the most important things people tend to think about is the pesticides. Many people choose to grow their own vegetables and fruits simply because they know the amount of pesticides that have been put on the foods they are eating.

It does no one any good to grow their own plants if they are just going to cover them with the same pesticides that are used in commercial growing. The great thing about hydroponics is that you do not have to use any pesticides. Many hydroponics systems are indoors, which prevents all pests that come from the soil and all disease. Even for those systems that are kept outside, there is no need for pesticides because since there is no dirt for the bugs and other pests to hide in, they leave the plants alone.

Another important factor that both those using hydroponics systems and traditional methods have to take into consideration is the impact of the fertilizer we are using. When you place fertilizer on your plants in a traditional garden, it does not do a lot of good. We have already talked about how the soil is depleted of nutrients, but many people think that placing fertilizer on the ground is going to help the plants absorb the nutrients they need but that really is not true. Most of the nutrients from the fertilizer get washed away with watering or rain and one of the biggest downsides to using fertilizer on your traditional garden is that you do not have any idea what nutrients you are giving to your plants.

On the other hand, when you use hydroponics, with fertilizers or nutrient rich solutions, you know that your plants are getting balanced nutrients. This nutrient rich solution is going to be washed over your root's day after day and one of the really great things about the solution is that it can be poured over plants that are in the ground each time you change your water and solution.

One of the things that many people do not like about hydroponics systems is that some of them do require extra energy. Of course, traditional gardening uses the light and the energy of the sun, but when you have a hydroponics system, whether indoors or out, you are going to use more electricity. You will need to use electricity for your pumps, your lights, your timers, and many of the other parts of your system. You have to weigh the positives and the negatives when it comes to deciding to use a hydroponics system and determine if using that extra amount of electricity is worth it for you. Another topic that many people want to know about concerning hydroponics versus traditional farming is the amount of water that is used. Many people would wrongly assume that traditional gardening uses the lowest amount of water, but the truth is that traditional gardening uses more water than hydroponics systems.

Water is used over and over again in a hydroponics system, which means using 90% less water than traditional gardening does. Hydroponics is a great way for you to grow your plants in a drought or in the desert where the conditions just do not support traditional farming.

Traditional farming is highly reliant upon the rain, which can lead to many issues.

When there is a drought, it can lead to the plants simply drying out and as it was here just last year, when there is a lot of flooding, plants tend to just wash away.

Traditional farming depends a lot on the land as well. This means that if you are like me and you have a large amount of land that is nothing but a rocky mess, you are not able to grow a traditional garden.

Hydroponics systems, however, do not rely on rain (unless, you are using the rainwater to fill your reservoir), the outside weather, or the conditions of the soil. If you put all of this together, it means that anyone can grow a garden, not just those in the Midwest with large front yards and a good amount of rainfall.

Hydroponics also outweighs traditional farming when it comes to bringing in the bacon. Because the plants grow at least twice as fast in a hydroponics system as they would in a traditional garden, you are going to yield more fruits and vegetables. You are also going to be growing very healthy fruits and vegetables, which is what people are looking for today. If you compare the two, traditional farming and hydroponics farming, you will quickly see that hydroponics wins out every time.

Chapter 7: The Best Plants for Hydroponic Gardening

First of all, it is necessary to know that cuttings rooted in water are ideal for starting hydroculture because, for them, it is much easier to adapt to the expanded clay substrate since it is mainly composed of water.

If you want to start with the cultivation of hydroculture plants, there is a great variety to choose from. If you are a lover of aromatic herbs, the rosemary plant is perfect for growing in hydroculture if you start from cutting; otherwise, you can choose other types of ornamental and very decorative plants, such as Ficus, Calathea, Pothos, Dracena, and Philodendron.

All plants characterized by leaves of tropical origin are well suited to hydroculture, such as the orchid and all those species that present a rapid development to the root system.

And what about flowering plants? In these cases, the most recommended species for home hydroculture are Hibiscus, Spathiphyllum, Kalanchoe, Anthurium, or Saintpaulia. Still, nothing prevents you from trying to cultivate other types of plants as well.

What about succulents? Succulents have a more complicated situation since they do not tolerate excess humidity. Therefore, the recommended species for hydroculture are aloe, succulent plants, and - as anticipated above - orchids.

Lettuce

Growing salad in hydroponics is elementary, much more than it might seem, even for those who start from scratch and approach the hydroponics world for the first time.

Once you have identified the variety of salad that best suits your needs and tastes, you must obtain the seeds that you will easily find online.

Then you will have to buy rock wool cubes (Rockwool) and net jars, a mini-green to store them in the warm, in a protected environment and with net pots, designed precisely for the needs of plants that are grown with hydroponic and aeroponic systems. Therefore, a small hydroponic or aeroponic system will be needed.

The salad seeds must be placed inside the moistened rock wool cubes (it is recommended not to insert more than five seeds for each cube) only with water and then placed inside the mini-greenhouse, at a temperature that can oscillate between 73°F (23°C) and 82°F (28°C).

One aspect to check - when using rock wool cubes - is the amount of water they absorb, because an excessive amount of liquid could cause the roots to rot and drown them. For this, it is always advisable to check the liquid levels present and possibly wring out the cubes to let out the excess water.

With the right amount of water and the ideal temperature, lettuce seeds will begin to germinate after about 48 hours.

When you see the first roots appearing from the rock wool cubes (both from the sides and the base), it means that the time has come to transfer the newly born seedlings to the special mesh pots, which will first be filled with expanded clay and then settled in the hydroponic system you have chosen (or aeroponic).

The seedlings inserted in the aeroponic system will then be fed with a special nutrient solution based on water and fertilizers to provide everything they need. It is vital to avoid any fertilizer during the germination phase and then start with a halved dose compared to what is recommended on the package.

Fertilizers for the cultivation of Hydroponic salad

By using suitable fertilizers and in the right dose, the roots of the lettuce seedlings are allowed to develop better and faster than they would use with a traditional cultivation system, also because - in this way - the roots can receive and assimilate nutrients faster.

Hydroponic salad: parameters to monitor

At this point, once the cultivation has started, it is appropriate to keep under control some fundamental values for the health and growth of each plant, such as the pH, which will determine the ability - by the cultivated plant - to correctly absorb the available nutrients.

In order for salad plants to absorb all nutrients correctly, the pH must be slightly acidic, and to ensure that it is always such, it is advisable to often monitor the situation with manual tests. For example, cheap and easy-to-use paper strips for pH testing can be used.

Tips and tricks for a perfect Hydroponic salad

To create a suitable and protected environment, it is recommended to repair and check the salad plants inside a grow box to make them grow well, healthily and faster, without weighing on the cost of the bill.

Among the advantages of using the grow box, there is undoubtedly that of being able to more easily control the temperature than a larger environment and, therefore, less controlled, better manage ventilation, ensure the right lighting (thanks to the reflective mylar sheet present inside the grow box which allows the light to be effectively propagated).

But when will you get your first salad crop?

Much depends on the variety chosen and cultivated, but - in general - it is possible to say that the time required varies between 4 weeks and 80 days. By choosing different varieties and managing the aeroponic system, you can have a fresh, tasty, and healthy salad at any time of the year.

To help grow, salad plants should be adequately lit: the best solution is to use HID discharge lamps or LEDs, but a good compromise can also be found by using fluorescent lamps.

To better manage the lighting of the salad plants, it is advisable to activate the lights for 12 hours a day, thus ensuring 12 hours of darkness.

Strawberries

Cross and delight of many professional and amateur growers, the strawberry is a problematic fruit, especially if grown out of season and in unsuitable environments. All difficulties are overcome, especially for those who choose the above-ground cultivation, better known as hydroponic cultivation.

The more than tested technique, especially in strawberry cultivation, offers more than exciting advantages:

- production is standardized;

- there is a considerable saving of energy and water, which is used more rationally;

- production is better in quality and quantity;

- the problem of diseases, molds, and pests that multiply on contact with the ground are entirely forgotten.

Those who choose the hydroponic technique also have the opportunity to produce strawberries in at least two different periods of the year: from October to December and throughout April and May.

If we also take into consideration that once planted, the plants begin to bear fruit after 45 days. It is well understood why this choice is shared by many growers and lovers of indoor cultivation.

Anyone who chooses to switch to this type of technique must first thoroughly wash the roots of their seedlings and insert them in a small pot that contains expanded clay or alchemy of vermiculite and perlite.

It is also essential to have a container that can hold at least 10 liters of water (for each seedling), better if impermeable to the passage of light to avoid the formation of algae and mushrooms.

Among the most popular hydroponic cultivation methods for strawberries, there is the one called NFT hydroponics: to make it simple with this system; it is possible to achieve a good circulation of all the nutrients that the roots need. Everything is automated thanks to the use of a timer that alternates between full and dry moments, essential for the roots to have the right oxygenation.

Obviously, it is essential to have the right fertilizer, which in this case, is composed of nitrogen and potassium and water with the correct pH, which should always be adjusted between 5.5 and 5.6. To make the job easier, there are active acidity regulators on the market.

Finally, you must have the right lighting, and in this case, the lamps for indoor cultivation will be a potent ally.

Once you start your strawberry cultivation, domestic or industrial, it is good to keep in mind that the plant must be regularly pruned: it is wrong not to cut excess leaves, especially before flowering. These will unnecessarily weaken the plant and could favor the creation of mushrooms that are particularly harmful to the future growth of strawberries.

Tomatoes

Quality and quantity with Hydroponic tomato cultivation

Tomato is a genuinely functional vegetable in hydroponic culture. It reacts very well to the so-called "soilless cultivation," this because it can easily adapt to different types of substrate and does not require demanding agronomic management.

In tomato hydroponics, multiple substrates can be used:

- Rock wool
- Peat
- Perlite
- Coconut fiber
- Compost

And with all, you can achieve magnificent results. The only precaution that must be paid in the hydroponic cultivation of tomatoes is the temperature. Indeed, excessive maxims could affect the floral drop and, therefore, on the quantity and quality of the product.

Kitchen herbs

The new home dream is to have a thousand and one aromatic herbs on the terrace or the balcony to flavor your dishes with a personal, fresh, and eco-friendly touch. This is why hydroponics has been so successful.

The Greeks already knew it, Francis Bacon spoke about it in 1627 and today hydroponics (literally the art of growing plants in water) is well appreciated in the industrial and domestic field.

The hydroponic cultivation of aromatic herbs has five remarkable qualities:

1. the yield of the product that is developed through indoor cultivation is better;

2. growth is faster;

3. the taste is more intense;

4. the cultivation technique is environmentally sustainable;

5. the water expenditure decreases drastically.

With hydroponic cultivation at home, it is possible to grow any aromatic plant, whether it is parsley, basil, thyme, rosemary, oregano. Still, you can also choose to grow lettuces, tomatoes, strawberries, and who knows what else.

In short, hydroponics allows at reduced costs and with a disarming simplicity to make your terrace or balcony a garden of wonders, a vertical garden, an urban oasis.

The roots of our aromatic seedlings will seek support on an inert substrate often made up of expanded clay, pralines, coconut fiber, or other similar materials. Of course, the irrigation that the plant receives must be rich in inorganic compounds that will be able to give it all the nutrients that generally come from the earth. Your cultivation of aromatic herbs will surely provide unparalleled satisfaction.

Orchids

Orchids lend themselves perfectly to hydroculture. They are, in fact, epiphytic plants (i.e., plants that naturally grow and live on other plants), and humid environments represent their ideal condition for growing well and in health.

The plant will develop its roots, which - with the growth and passage of time - will pass through the holes of the pot, to flow directly into the water. Different varieties of orchids can be grown in hydroculture, such as the best-known variety of Phalaenopsis, but also Cattleya, the Dendrobium variety, Paphiopedilum and Oncydium.

Chapter 8: Maintenance

Hydroponic gardens need to have the proper care and maintenance, or they will not produce healthy plants. Not only do they need to be constantly cleaned, but there are various maintenance checks that need to be carried out in order to make sure the system remains functioning correctly.

A faulty drain, or a leaky pipe or switch could do serious damage to a hydroponic garden as most of the systems rely on their equipment and parts to work smoothly.

Cleanliness

In order to stop the build-up of algae, mold, and fungus or to stop attracting pests, keep the growing room as clean as possible.

Equipment should be flushed and cleaned at least twice a month to maintain water levels, stop algae growth, and ensure that there are no pests lurking about the system.

In order to stop pests and various fungal growth, growers should always make sure their hands are clean. Hands should be kept washed especially after handling anything that was dirty or in contact with a harmful substance.

Do not let old fallen leaves, stems, fruit, produce or growing media or even pots or discarded trays lie around the growing areas. Rather throw out any debris or broken items, and wash and pack away any unused equipment.

Wash all equipment after use and only reuse a growing medium if it can be reused and it has been thoroughly washed and sterilized. In fact, all growing mediums, whether old or new, should be thoroughly washed before being used as not to contaminate the grow pots, grow trays, and the reservoir.

Keeping the growing area and equipment clean cuts down on the chances of infestation and development of frustrating diseases that are a nuisance to get rid of.

Nutrient Solution

The proper nutrient solution for the plant type and system type should be used at the correct ratio of solution to water.

Image result for hydroponic nutrient solution

Only use good quality nutrient solutions with an organic base. Advance nutrients are only required should there be a problem that needs to be fixed, such as a nutrient deficiency in a plant.

The nutrient solution balance should be checked on a regular basis especially is it is a recovery system where the solution is being continuously recycled.

Make sure that the solution is flushed and completely refreshed on a regular basis and that there is no salt buildup, since this is very acidic and toxic to the plants.

Watering

Watering is done in many different ways and is delivered to each of the hydroponic systems differently.

Make sure the water is always fresh and checked on a regular basis. Algae is a common problem, as is nutrient build up in the system. An oxygen pump should be installed in order to ensure the water is being well hydrated and to keep the water fresher for longer.

Water solutions can come from the tap, drain systems, or rain collection tanks.

Watering can be on a continuous flow basis or set by a timer that switches on and off at different intervals during the day.

If possible, a person should always have a backup water solution available in case of an emergency and their primary watering source is unavailable. Some plants are very sensitive to their watering schedule and even a few minute's downtime and a missed watering schedule can cause some damage.

Reservoir Temperature

The water in the reservoir should be around 65 to 75 degrees Fahrenheit, which is basic room temperature. Water that is either too hot or too cold can damage the plant's root systems and their leaves.

The reservoir should be topped off with water in order to keep pH and nutrient levels constant. Change out the water on a regular basis.

Humidity

Different plants and hydroponic systems need the humidity to be on different levels. There are thermometers that can measure the humidity and temperature to ensure that the plants are comfortable. Keeping an optimum level does not encourage the growth of unwanted diseases and fungi.

Make sure plants that love the hotter temperatures get enough humidity by giving them a regular misting spray. This will help to keep the humidity constant for the plants that do not like too much humidity.

Inspect the Equipment

The equipment should be thoroughly inspected on a regular basis.

There are a lot of things that can go wrong in a hydroponic system, especially with the equipment. And the best way to troubleshoot is to try to avoid as many equipment malfunctions as possible.

The best way to inspect equipment it to keep the entire system in mind. When doing the inspection start at one point and work your way through your system.

Start with the reservoir and all the systems that are dependent on it.

- Water feeding pipe

  o   This should be thoroughly checked for crimps that may not be feeding the solution correctly.

- Nutrients build up in the pipes so they may need a thorough flushing out or replacing.
- Check for any blockages in the pipe.
- Check for any holes or leaks that could deter the flow of water pressure in the pipe.
- Check for any algae or mold that may be growing in or around the pipe.
- Determine if it may be time to replace the hoses.
- Give them a good cleaning if they are still viable.

* Nozzles and hoses

- Check the nozzles that feed the root systems, sprinklers, or misting systems.
- When last were they changed?
- Check for blockages or leakage.
- Check any joins and washers for leaks.
- Check for sediment build up, algae, or mold growing in or around these attachments.
- Give them a good cleaning if they are still usable.

* Drain siphons and hoses

- Check the drainpipes for blockages
- When last were they replaced?
- Check for leaks.
- Check for algae or mold growing in or around these pipes.
- They may need to have a good cleaning as part of the system maintenance.

- **Check the reservoir water pump**
- Test the pump
- Make sure it is still working correctly and pumping the water at the optimum flow.
- Check that all pump attachments are not leaking air.

- **Check the reservoir**
- Check that there is no build-up, algae, or mold growing on the reservoir.
- Check for any leaks.
- Make sure the water is at the optimum temperature for the hydroponic system and plants.

- Check that any air pumps are functioning correctly and adequately oxygenating the tank.
- Make sure any oxygen stones do not have unwanted algae or mold growth on them

- **Growing trays**

- Make sure the growing tray(s) do not have any leaks in them.
- Make sure the growing tray(s) are clean and have not unwanted algae or mold growing on them.
- Clean off any nutrient build up and make sure the trays are clean.
- For a closed system, the trays must be given thorough flushing out.

- **Growing pots**

- Check that each of the pots is still intact and not broken.
- Replace any that are not functioning correctly.
- Make sure any growing medium is clean and does not have any unwanted algae or mold growing on them that could upset the plant's natural balance.

- Lighting equipment
    - Check that the bulbs are still functioning correctly.
    - Check that the lighting is still adequate for the environment.
    - Check the timers are working correctly.
    - Clean any residue off the lighting system.

Temperature

- Make sure that any thermostat is working correctly, and that room temperature is normal.
- Check that the humidity is correct for the growing environment.
- Check both the temperature and humidity thermometers to ensure that they are still working correctly.

Ventilation

- Make sure that there is adequate ventilation in the growing room.
- Not enough ventilation can cause mold.
- Check that all fans and cooling systems are working correctly.

- Support Systems

o   Check that any hanging supports for the plants are working without causing the plant or system any undue stress.

o   Make sure that the environment in which the hydroponic system is housed offers the correct infrastructure for the system to function correctly.

o   Make sure the plants are all supported and planted correctly to ensure a successful infrastructure.

Tools

o   Are all the gardening tools in working order?

o   Are they cleaned?

o   Are there any that may need to be replaced?

Look at Your Plants

Make sure you keep a vigilant check on your growing plants. Measure their growth rate, root growth and when they are ready to harvest.

This gives a person a good measure of how the next batch should perform and something by which to determine if the growing medium, solution, or systems structure may need to be changed or optimized.

The plants must also be checked to make sure they are getting enough nutrients, they are growing as they should, and there are no pests or other infestations. A lot of growing problems and deficiencies can be caused by various infestations. Some are easy to spot, others may take more of an experienced eye, but as a gardener gets to know their plants they will come to instinctively know when something is wrong.

Look for the signs in seedlings such as slow growth, looking sad and droopy, white fluffy stuff growing on the leaves, etc.

Take the time to look over the plants; do not just rush through it. If there are a lot of plants to look over, break them and do a revolving sweep of one on this day, and the next on another.

If there is an outbreak, you will need to go through the entire growing area right away.

Spending time with the plants in a hydroponic environment can also be quite good for the mind and spirit. Plants and running water are rather therapeutic and can reduce stress, anxiety and ease tension.

Change One Thing at a Time

If you are wanting to change or expand your system, do not try and do it all at once.

Choose to change, switch it around, or upgrade and start with that.

Before rushing out and buying expensive parts, why not try a bit of DIY and try to make it yourself. Or at least look around to see what you have available before rushing off to spend more money on an item you do not really need.

Hydroponic systems are not only flexible and versatile in what they can grow or how they deliver their solutions, but they can also be easily adapted to suit the grower's needs and lifestyle.

There are so many great DIY ideas on how to create the perfect hydroponic garden online these days that it is well worth a try. The money you save building the system yourself can be better spent on plants, growing media, or nutrient solutions.

In order to keep a system simple and working for you, think carefully about an upgrade or addition. Plot it out and then work through one at a time getting that part right before moving on to the next.

Chapter 9: The Myths and Errors to Avoid

Our time together has almost come to a close. Before you go out and get going on your own garden, let us take the time to look at some of the mistakes and myths that pop up frequently in discussions on hydroponic gardening. By digging through the myths to find the truth and learning from the mistakes of those that came before us, we are able to benefit from the knowledge and avoid making the same mistakes ourselves.

Mistake: Hard-to-Use Setups

When you are setting up your hydroponic garden, it is important that you consider how hard it will be to use. Are you going to have a difficult time reaching the plants in the back because you put the garden up against a wall? Are you going to bump into the lights every time you try to tend the bed because the space is too small and cramped?

When you are setting up your garden it is important that you consider issues such as the physical space in which it will sit. You want to make sure that you can get to all your plants without a struggle. If you're knocking over lights or throwing your back out to reach plants, then the setup isn't going to be a very good one. Chances are you are going to end up breaking something or neglecting it. Consider the ways in which you move through the garden space; make sure that you are able to reach everything.

You also want to make sure that you are able to get to your reservoir easily. While it may be tempting just to rest the grow tray on top of the reservoir, consider how this might cause issues when it comes time to switch the nutrient solution. Will you have somewhere to place the grow tray while you have to mess around with the reservoir? If not, then how did you plan to do it?

Myth: Hydroponic Gardens Are Only for Illegal Substances

It seems that any time hydroponics pop up in the news it is in relation to some illegal grow operation that has been busted by the police. This has led to a stigma around hydroponics, one which it really doesn't deserve. Just because it happens that a lot of illegal growers use hydroponic setups, it doesn't mean that hydroponics is used just for illegal purposes.

As we saw above, we went an entire book looking at hydroponics and never once did we mention any drugs. We looked at how hydroponics will help our herb gardens to produce 30% more aromatic oils. We talked about vegetables and fruits. Never once did we speak about illegal substances.

This is because hydroponics is a system for growing plants. Those plants don't need to be illegal. They can be, yes. But they can also be the garden veggies you serve in a salad. Hydroponics is just a great system for growing plants, and it is a system that you can run from inside your house, which means that you can hide your garden easily. But hydroponics itself is not illegal, it does not mean that you are taking part in illegal activities and this particular myth should be put to rest already.

Mistake: Choosing the Wrong Crops for Your Climate

You hear about a new crop on one of the gardening sites you check online. It sounds like it could be a lot of fun to grow, some kind of berry you never heard of before and people say it does great in a hydroponic setup. You order some seeds, plant it and it grows but it just doesn't give the results you wanted. Looking to see what goes wrong, you do some more Googling on the plant and you realize it needs to be in a super-hot, arid environment. And you're living through the coldest winter of your life.

Different plants want different climates, and nothing will be more disappointing than trying to grow a plant that just doesn't like the climate you can offer. We should always do our research on the plants that we want to grow. We can do this easily with Google or by going into our local hydroponic store to speak to the staff.

Myth: Hydroponics Have to be Done Indoors

We've spoken a lot about indoor hydroponics. This was a choice to highlight the fact that we can raise hydroponics indoors. There any many people out there who don't have access to an outside plot in which to start a garden. Most people that live in an apartment building have at best a balcony and many don't even have that much. Being that you can have an indoor garden, hydroponics offers a way for more people to get into gardening.

But this doesn't mean that you can't have an outdoor hydroponic garden. When we raise our gardens indoors, we are able to control the seasons and really take an active role in maintaining the humidity and temperature, how long the grow lights are on and much more. If we grow outdoors, then we can save money on grow lights by using the sun but we also open our garden up to more risk from pests and disease. However, hydroponics can be done anywhere that you want.

Mistake: Picking the Wrong Plants for Your Setup

This could also be called "Not Doing Your Research." Like picking plants that match your climate, you are also going to want to make sure you pick plants that will work well in your setup. Some plants work better in different systems. Some want less water; some want slower draining and others want more water and others yet want faster draining.

It is important that you research the plants that you want to put in your garden. There are hundreds upon hundreds of websites jam-packed with information about every plant you could consider growing. They will tell you the pH and EC levels for the plant, how hot they like their environment, how much water they want and what type of hydroponic setup is best for them. We looked at a handful throughout, but there is no way we could have covered all of them. But Google is your friend.

So, make sure you do your research and plan out your garden. Preparing yourself with information will avoid costly mistakes. Not only does it cost to grow but there is also a time cost and you will lose weeks before you realize that growing that one plant is a losing battle.

Myth: Hydroponics is Super Expensive

This myth has good reason to be around. The truth is that hydroponics can be expensive. Can be. But just because it can be doesn't mean that it always is. When you head to the hydroponic store and look at all the prices and get talked into buying more than you really needed, then it is going to be expensive. But like many hobbies, it depends on how serious you want to take it and you can always start slow.

There are a ton of ways to cut down costs when beginning your garden. Searching online you can find hundreds of do-it-yourself guides to starting a hydroponic setup. These offer great ways to try out hydroponic gardening for the new grower. You can get your hands dirty and really see if it is something that you enjoy before you go spending a lot of money. Speaking of spending a lot of money.

Mistake: Scaling Up the Operation Too Early

Starting off too big can be a terrible mistake. For one, it means sinking a lot of money into growing right out the gate. Before you do this, you should at least have some experience with hydroponics. Another big issue is that until you have some experience you don't actually know how to best care for your garden and every step in the operation cycle is going to be a learning experience. This isn't bad when we start small but starting bigger means any mistakes, we make along the way are going to cost us that much more.

You should start slow and learn the ropes. As you go along you can buy more expensive equipment as you figure out what equipment you actually need and what equipment works best with your style of growing. As you learn the way your plants take to the system, get a feel for how they grow in your setup, then you can begin to expand. You can start to add in another grow tray, maybe two. But add slowly, take your time and make sure you have a good grasp of how to run a small garden before you jump into a large one. You can always get there, but patience will help save you from some truly devastating mistakes along the way. It's one thing to mess up one grow tray, it's another to mess up a dozen.

Myth: Hydroponics is Unnatural

What happened to just stick a plant in the ground and letting it grow? Hydroponics seems like a lot of work to do the same thing. The plants come out bigger, too. Seems like there must be something unnatural going on here. It must be all those chemicals used in the solution.

Of course, this myth is just silly. We are growing plants and using natural mix in our grow trays. We mix together a nutrient solution, but all of these are natural nutrients that the plants take from the Earth anyway. Hydroponics is just a system of growing. We grow healthy plants the same as any gardener tries to. There are no gross chemicals being used to give us better growth than soil. All we are doing is using the natural desires of the plant to provide it with the most comfortable growing experience we can.

Mistake: Not Maintaining Your Garden

I know, I know. You've heard this one before. But it is the number one mistake that new growers make and so we are going to speak about it one last time. The fact is that maintaining your garden doesn't just mean changing the water. It doesn't just mean we look at the garden when the plants look ill and infected and get to work. Maintaining our gardens is a commitment that any gardener has to honor.

Something spill? Better wipe that up. There's dead plant matter in your grow tray or on the floor around your setup? Best clean that up and get rid of it. Infestations and infections love to grow in these conditions. So, check your plants, test the water, clean up the beds and show them a little love. You wouldn't let your dog sleep in its own waste, so why would you let your plants? Maintaining your garden is the most important thing you can do as a new grower.

Treat your plants right.

Mistake: Forgetting to Have Fun

If you are growing because you want to sell your crops, that's a fine reason to do it. But try to have fun. For many, this is an enjoyable hobby and brings them a lot of peace.

Chapter 10: Hydroponics vs. Soil Gardening

Arguments have always abounded on which is better between soil gardening and hydroponic gardening. Some people are of the opinion that soil gardening beats hydroponic gardening, while some others argue that hydroponic gardening is definitely better than soil gardening.

So, which do we believe?

Soil Gardening

Soil gardening, as you know, is more affordable because the equipment needed are just simple tools and types of machinery, nothing ambiguous. Plus, typically, you do not need to adjust so much about the soil as it does this itself, using its environment as a gage. Since plants will naturally grow on soil, it is only natural for the soil to be gentle on plants. Overall, soil gardening seems so much easier than hydroponics, what is not to love?

Well, those are only the good sides; would you be able to deal with the bad sides?

First off, it takes longer for plants to grow in the soil. You will also notice defects late because it takes longer for these defects to become visible. What this means is that the defects would have done so much damage before they are finally noticed, ultimately making the recovery of the plants difficult and longer. This could take its toll on your money and your time.

Then, at the beginning of your plant's growth in the soil, it will require all the attention and patience as it is still tender and quite vulnerable.

You also have to deal with preventing bugs from feasting on your plants. This is an almost impossible feat, and it's best to stick with hydroponics if you can't deal with the bugs.

Hydroponic Gardening

In hydroponic gardening, you have total control over the nutrient supply provided to your plants. This will help minimize problems that usually develop from an inadequate nutrient supply in the soil.

You also skip so much growing time and get to harvest really quick because the nutrients come directly to your plants and your plants do not expend so much time and energy in search of nutrients, as is the case in soil gardening. They, therefore, spend most of the time and energy on their growth, which ends up happening fast. As a matter of fact, a plant grown hydroponically under same conditions as one grown in the soil can grow fifty percent faster.

Plus, since your plants grow faster when grown hydroponically, you get to identify defects on time and fix them right on time.

At this point, I bet you now see just how much more beneficial hydroponics gardening is, and this is just the introduction!

Is hydroponic gardening even healthy?

The nutrients supplied in a hydroponic system are not in any way different from the one in the soil; it is gotten from mineral salts. What is different in the nutrient supply is, as I mentioned, that the roots of plants grown in the soil have to go in search of nutrients; that is what makes their root systems so large. Plants grown hydroponically do not have to do this, because the nutrients go directly to the roots and in the right amount. This lets the plant spend less time growing root systems and more time growing leaves and stems.

What you get as a result is strong and healthy plants.

Gradually, more commercial growers are starting to embrace hydroponic gardening over soil gardening, because it is amazing that you can control the supply of nutrients to your plants and conserve space. This ultimately boosts yield and profit.

Plants that are grown hydroponically are also not as susceptible to diseases and pests as plants grown on the soil, because of how vigorous they are. The plants possess anti-pest and anti-fungal buffers that keep them protected. This means less money spent on fertilizers, fungicides and pesticides and more safe foods, as the consumption of chemical-ridden plants no longer becomes an issue. Plants that have been sprayed with fungicides and other chemicals have detrimental effects on the health and the practice is worth doing away with.

Worthy of note is how much better hydroponic system is for the preservation of the environment. Since water circulates throughout the system, it does not get sucked into the ground or evaporate quickly. So far, hydroponics has done so much for modern day agriculture and contributed to the supply of fresh plants that are free from blemish.

This is a summary that I am sure already convinced you to consider hydroponic gardening. But just in case you are not as certain yet, we will get into the details immediately.

Why You Should Pick Hydroponic Gardening Over Soil Gardening

You Produce Chemical-Free Plants

When the soil is taken out of the equation, this translates to less pests and diseases to deal with. Plants grown hydroponically are not as susceptible to diseases and pests because of the absence of soil and how healthy they are. Pests tend to gravitate towards weaker plants and there are hardly weak plants in the hydroponic system, making pest infestations almost impossible. This in turn means that there is little or no need for fungicides and pesticides. In the end, you get plants that are not laden with toxic and unhealthy chemicals.

Saves Space

Since plants grown hydroponically rarely have bulky roots because they do not have to go in search of nutrients, you can grow more plants in smaller spaces. These plants will thrive; they have everything they need provided in the nutrient solution that is ideally measured and supplied. Planting your crops closely together rewards you with space saving.

Saves Water

So much water is saved in the hydroponic gardening system. In the traditional soil garden system, large volumes of water are expended in watering the plants, this is done so that a significant part of the water gets absorbed by the soil and sucked up by the roots of the plants. Unfortunately, this system isn't such a great one because water ends up getting wasted.

How?

First off, after a good amount is poured out into the soil, only a reasonable amount gets to the root of the plant. The rest of the water either goes further down in the soil or evaporates. Whereas, in the hydroponic garden system, a recirculating nutrient reservoir is employed. Plant roots only take up some of the water at a time, the rest of the water is preserved for later. This preserved water in the reservoir is covered to ensure no evaporation occurs and water cannot seep through the bottom.

With this system, the amount of water that has gone into watering a plant in one day could be used for several weeks in the hydroponic system. So much water saving!

Location

Unlike in the soil gardening where you have to worry about location and external environment hospitability, the case is different in hydroponic gardening. As I mentioned before, everything in the hydroponic system is under your control, you are the boss. As a result, you would not have to worry a lot about location (you can't do it anywhere); first because you do not even need so much space and secondly, you can control the external environment of the plant. Since hydroponic systems do not require so much space and strategic locations, you can set up your hydroponic garden in urban areas that have little space without worrying. You can also grow your plants close to the market, thus, reducing transportation costs. As regards controlling the external environment of the plants, you are in charge of the nutrient supply and the light. There are artificial lights you can use when there is little or no access to sunlight for whatever reason. The seasons have no effect whatsoever on the hydroponically grown plants because you control the environment, not the seasons. This means you can grow a plant in a season when it is difficult to grow it, this earns you more profit.

Impressive Growth of Plants

In soil gardening, plants take so much time and energy developing root systems for searching for nutrients, water and oxygen. As a result, they do not grow as fast because not as much time and energy is geared towards developing the leaves, stem, and most importantly, fruit.

On the other hand, plants grown hydroponically get to grow much faster because they have all of the nutrients, oxygen and water right at their roots (I would say at their fingertips if they had fingers, but you get the point). Since they don't have to do so much searching for nutrients, oxygen and water, they can spend all their time growing. This way, they're grown in short periods, which means you get to have more growth cycles for other plants in a given time. Plus, the plants also grow bigger. As a result, you get more yields. For emphasis, studies confirm that hydroponically grown plants tend to grow up to fifty percent faster and bigger than soil grown plants.

Control

Even though this has been said a lot in passing while explaining other points, this is a point too. In the soil gardening system, it is difficult to control a number of things, like amount of water the plants get, amount of nutrients gotten by the plants, the nutrient make-up of the soil, pests, diseases, pH, etc.

In the hydroponic system, all these factors are easily regulated so you do not have to beat your head. You call the shots over what nutrients and how much your plants get, how much water your plants get and how much is preserved, the pH of the oxygenated solution, the lighting and your plants are protected from pests and diseases.

No Weeding/Digging

This is good news for some. Unlike in the conventional gardening system with soils where you have to spend so much time on dirt, taking out weeds, building mounds and the likes, there is no such thing in hydroponics. Since you are not dealing with soil, lots of soil issues give way, one of which is weeds. It is annoyingly time-consuming to spend ages doing this. With hydroponics, this problem is solved.

Cleanliness

No soil means there would be no problems. With soil comes all the unpleasant stuff like parasites, weeds, pests and dirt. In the hydroponic system, you will not have to deal with this mess. You can garden without getting yourself dirty. Hydroponics is obviously the cleaner choice!

Cost

At first, the initial cost of hydroponics can look like a huge disadvantage. However, as time goes on, the ground pretty much levels up.

How do I mean?

It is much cheaper to set up a soil garden than a hydroponic system. However, along the line, soil gardening starts to cost more. Money is spent on things like fertilizers, herbicides, pesticides, fungicides, and water.

Little or No Diseases and Pests

as I said before, taking the soil out of the equation means that you would not have to deal with pests and diseases as much any longer. In the hydroponic system where a liquid media is used, it is almost impossible for pests to find their way to the plants and cause harm, it is also impossible to have to deal with soil-borne diseases.

Chapter 11: Making Money from Your Greenhouse

If you have a successful greenhouse that grows beautiful plants and flowers, why not consider making some money from your hobby?

You might not have ever thought about your hobby as a profitable business, but if you have at least a little bit of extra time and patience, you can actually make quite a nice income from your greenhouse. Find Your Niche For any grower to be successful, they need to be aware of and be able to make use of current niches and trends in the growing market. The advantage of greenhouse growing is that you can have an extended season of growth that other more natural growers would not have.

This means that you can grow special flowers, fruits, and veggies that would not normally be available to others much later in the year.

There is always a market for certain crops, especially when they begin to become out of season, so this creates an immediate cash crop for you to make money. Special fall flowers such as Dwarf Snapdragons are much sought after by late fall, and typically only greenhouse growers can meet the demand that most retailers need. But along with extending the growing time for rare flowers and produce, in finding your niche, you need to find out what kind of production makes the most money.

Often enough, there are best sellers in the market, such as tomatoes and jalapeno peppers, and the popular demand may vary based upon your geographical area. As soon as you find your niche, you can begin to make a whole lot of money in the process.

Becoming a Business One of the first things you should do before you start conducting business is become a business.

This means getting a business name, typically done through your county clerk's office. Most who start a small business use a Doing Business as or Assumed Name; this means that income from your business is the same as income from any other place.

You add up your income and subtract your expenses and report the final amount on your tax return at the end of the year. Unless you plan on opening a retail flower store, you probably don't need to collect taxes from your customers as you would be considered a wholesaler.

However, if your business grows and you're concerned about your need to collect taxes, you can probably quickly speak to a CPA over the phone and ask. Usually, applying for a tax ID is very easy and probably done at your county clerk's office as well. These certificates - your Assumed Name and tax ID - are typically very affordable, usually less than twenty dollars each.

Don't hesitate to call your county clerk's office first if you want to be sure your chosen business name isn't already taken or aren't sure which certificate is right for you. You can probably also check online as many counties have their own website where you can run off the forms you need and can find out the charge. Once you have your business certificates, you can open a commercial checking account at just about any bank and may also want to check to see if you can reserve a website name that is at least close to your business name. Important:

When coming up with a business name, you can, of course, have it a bit whimsical; people often assume a greenhouse or flower shop has a bit of whimsy or creativity. Just make sure that it still sounds professional and is easy to remember and spell so that potential customers can remember it and find it again very easily. For instance, you might want to avoid "Debbie's Total Supply of Flowers and Plants from Her Own Greenhouse to Your Table" since it's incredibly long and wordy, but "Deb's Greenhouse and Flower Supply" is much easier to remember! Finding Customers So how to find customers, and what type of items should you sell? Here are some things you want to consider.

First, make sure your gardening is reliable and that you can grow enough of an inventory on a regular basis so that your customers won't be disappointed.

Being able to produce one flowering lily plant is all well and good, but if you want actually to make money from your business, you're going to need to produce beautiful flowers regularly.

This will, of course, mean being very attentive to your greenhouse and your plants.

No one wants to buy their flowers from someone who comes through with deliveries only when they can.

Yes, you'll lose some flowers here and there and, of course, can't always count on how many flowers you can actually grow, but to be successful with your business, you're going to need to have a pretty reliable idea of what you can and cannot deliver. Next, you'll need to consider what type of customers you can support with your inventory.

Flower shops sometimes have their own greenhouse for their supply, and supermarkets may have a floral shop, but because of how many flowers they need, they may want to deal only with a large commercial greenhouse facility. However, there are many other possibilities when it comes to customers that you can support. For example: Do you have any mini markets or corner stores near your home that sell a small number of flowers?

Even if you don't see them selling flowers now if you were to talk to the manager or owner of the store, you might be able to convince them to carry a small inventory.

Restaurants sometimes want fresh flowers for their tables.

You may be able to speak to a manager about providing carnations or other colorful blooms for their dining area or décor.

Retirement communities also sometimes have fresh flowers on their dining tables; you may be able to provide these for them regularly.

Businesses often give flowers to their employees on secretary's day or when someone has had a baby or other occasion. If you're priced cheaper than large, national florists, you may be able to provide for local businesses when the occasion calls for it.

Weddings, of course, are big business for many florists.

While you may not be ready to supply to very large weddings on a moment's notice, if you spread the word among your friends and relatives, you might find that someone you know is interested in working with you, especially if your costs are lower than national florists.

Many brides today are looking to save money in any way they can, so they may be happy to simply choose from the flowers you have available.

Your friends and family too may want to see what flowers you have available on special days and occasions. They may check with you for anniversaries, birthdays, and holidays.

Very often, getting the word out there among your friends and family and local businesses is all that's needed to get your first order, which in turn can lead to so many other orders down the road! Some Important Considerations Before you just run out and start talking to those retirement home managers and restaurant owners, consider some of the following points: Consider getting a website even if you don't plan on selling online.

A website is actually a great marketing tool because potential customers will often bookmark your site and visit again when they're ready to purchase. A website address is often easier to remember than a phone number, so customers might visit your site looking for your actual contact information.

Websites are usually very affordable if you just need a few pages with your contact info and a few photos of your product. Most places that purchase flowers from you may expect some type of special packaging.

For example, that corner market might be interested in purchasing single blooms that they keep by the cash register for one-at-a-time purchases.

However, these blooms are usually wrapped in cellophane and may have new ferns or baby's breath inside. Be prepared with these extra materials and for the wrapping involved; don't just show up with an armful of single blossoms.

Stores may also expect you to provide the large vase that these flowers are kept in near the register. View this as a marketing opportunity; put a card with your business name and phone number or website address on the front of it.

Get to know the accessories you need for many of your products. If you're going to provide bridal bouquets, you'll need the little handles they fit into. Boutonnieres for groomsmen usually are attached with a pin.

That retirement community may also ask you to provide vases. Shop for wholesale items online so you can purchase these things very cheaply. If you're very dedicated about making this greenhouse into a successful business, take a flower arranging class.

Putting together bouquets and arrangements is usually part art but part science.

Sometimes certain colors or sizes of flowers are just too busy or may look overdone when used together.

At the very least, study bouquets you see online and practice some on your own before trying to sell them to a customer.

Another thing you might want to consider about getting customers and selling is to have some marketing material available. At the very least, you should have professional business cards made up so that when you call upon potential customers, you have something you can leave with them, so they have your contact info handy.

You might also be able to make up a flyer or brochure with some featured products. If you can't do this on your own, you can easily hire someone with a marketing degree to do this for you; chances are you might even have a friend with some talent that can easily design some business cards or marketing material.

Any nearby office supply center can probably print these things out for a very affordable price. Calculate Your Profit Window In order to be successful with your greenhouse, you need to assess just how profitable the enterprise will be.

This means that you need to calculate your potential profit window in advance. First, you need to take into consideration how much money you will have to put into the greenhouse project. If it is just a small amount of money, you can set aside the small amount you may need; if it is a larger amount, you can then plan for that also.

Chapter 12: Tips, Tricks, and Hacks to Always Grow Healthy Plants in Your Garden

A hydroponic garden comes with several advantages, and one that stands out, is the increased growth rate. With the proper set up. Plants would mature faster and grow even faster than plants grown with soil. One of the reason plants in a hydroponic system grows so fast is because they do not have to work to get nutrients. The root system in a hydroponic system no matter how small will focus more on growing upwards instead of expanding the roots system downwards. All these movements are made possible due to controlled systems and because the systems are enclosed and managed properly, there is a careful control of nutrient solution, pH level and temperature. In hydroponics, there is less evaporation when compared to soil farming because of the enclosed system.

There are risks with using a hydroponics system, but one way to manage these risks is by proper maintenance. Check your system regularly. A broken or faulty pump could kill the plants, so proper maintenance of tools should not be overemphasized. Constant checks of the entire system save time and increases productivity. Not being cut unawares, being prepared always or at most times is an easy but not adhered to tip having healthy plants in a hydroponics garden.

Hydroponics systems require constant attention and care, and this can be tedious. It requires constant supervision of temperature, light, heat, PH level and this can take a toll on the gardener, and there is also the issue of forgetting to do things at an allocated time. Using a timer helps to regulate time and allows for running an organized system. Taking away the tedious process of checking the time regularly. Some tools and equipment have timers attached to them or specifically for them. The lights for example, some plants require long periods of exposure to light, others require shorter periods of exposure to light and some require a period of darkness in certain proportions, there are also times when the intensity of the light should be reduced, this chore can be made by using a timer, a timer that works with lighting. Having a timer or equipment with timers is a trick that makes things easy for gardeners. Small hydroponics systems may not need timers, especially when there are a few plants growing, this can easily be managed. Using a timer is extremely beneficial to certain hydroponics system and can be done without in some.

Generally, having a timer makes hydroponics gardening easy.

Most people have hydroponic gardens for different reasons, as hobbies, as a profession, for experiments, and some just to have access to healthy vegetables and fruits. It is good to know that with hydroponics you can grow almost plant. Some plants require more professional skill than others, while some can be grown with basic knowledge of hydroponics. Plants grown in a hydroponics system, that do very well and yield great results in fruit and flowers, Tomatoes, lettuce, spinach, basil, cucumbers, pepper, strawberry amongst many other. Knowing your plant and plant needs is a trick to growing healthy plant in a hydroponic system.

Knowing the plant, it nutritional needs, its light needs, its required temperature and the growth medium, helps saves time, money and manpower. For example, for beginners starting your hydroponics garden with growing Tomatoes may proof a bit difficult even though they are ideal for a hydroponics garden, they require a small ground space to grow and can be controlled to grow for as high as the grower wants, planting tomatoes should be done after practice with other vegetables that are easier to grow, because it requires a more controlled environment and less attention than a couple of other vegetables like Lettuce. Lettuce is one of the top plants to grow in a hydroponic garden especially for beginners because it requires less space and very little attention and in few weeks of planting, harvest can be ready. Peppers grows a bit like tomatoes they need regular observations and constant supervision, the only difference is the temperature and lighting needs of peppers, raising nighttime temperature and reducing day time temperatures is better for the peppers, they tend to produce better and healthier fruits that way. Spinaches, like the lettuce and most vegetables grow well in a hydroponic system, in fact they are fast growing in a hydroponic system. Strawberries thrives in a hydroponic system. They grow bigger than in the soil. They produce bigger fruits, blueberries, as well.

A trick to always remember is knowing your plant and your plant needs.

Lighting is another unavoidable aspect of hydroponics gardening, when plants have inadequate or the wrong type of lighting they can be stunted. Lighting tips includes; control the intensity of the light the plants receive by carefully selecting the watts of the bulb, the watts suit your plants intensity needs. The most common bulb watts go from 400-600watts. Regulate the amount of light the plants receive, grow plants that have the same or almost the same light needs together. They also require rest periods from light, just like the human body needs rest from the metabolic processes, plants also need rest for proper functioning and good growth rate. Again, a timer is a good trick to invest in especially with lights. In picking lights for your system, picking two of the three different lights is an amazing idea, because the systems may need different things at different stages of plant growth. The fluorescents are good and more efficient than the incandescent bulbs, they produce a lot of lights and use less electricity but when it comes to larger plants their intensity hardly penetrates them. So, know what light properties would be great for your plant. The distance between the plants and the light also affects growth because some lights are stronger than the other. The fluorescents can be placed close to the plants a distance of about 15cm from the plants is acceptable and wouldn't hurt plant health, for the high intensity discharge (HID) which is stronger than the fluorescents, a distance of about 50cm from the plant should be maintained to prevent harming the plants. The light emission diode is more expensive, but if you are thing long term, it is the light for you. It saves cost in the long run, because the bulbs can last for years and even a decade.

Another trick notable of remembering is the distance between the light and the plant to prevent harm, use a measuring tape if necessary.

A couple of people consider flushing optional, but a healthy hydroponics garden needs this action. Flushing is the removal of salt precipitate and other debris from the growth medium, pipes, pumps and every other part of the system. A good tip is doing this right before harvesting because it improves the flavor of your crops. It is also good to do this every time the nutrient solution is replaced. A trick to keep your plants looking healthy, every time the plants shows any signs of distress, Flushing might just be what the system needs. Flushing removes algae. There are flushing agents sold in hydroponics store, choose whichever is peculiar to your plants flushing needs.

A good trick to clean up clogged systems is by flushing more than once. Certain discoloration like brown spots on leaves or curled leaves maybe as a result of excess salt in the plants and flushing at that point is unavoidable to avoid the death of the plants.

Other tips and tricks to know when running a hydroponic system:

Plant in Lay-Out Pattern

The use of layouts in rows and columns helps organize the plants in a simple layout which makes it easier for the gardener to apply weedicides, water, and easily access the growth rate of his or her plants. It also allows him or her to adopt principles of 'shifting cultivation' and 'bush fallowing', allowing a certain allocated portion of the soil rest, while another is being cultivated. Essentially a layout pattern enables the user to have a healthy soil, and in turn, have a healthy yield of plants. But an important word of caution, the plants should not be spaced so tightly, because plants generally do not reach their full size when crowded.

Employ the Use of a Vertical Support System or a Trellis System

A vertical support system is essential for the growth of hydroponic plants, it's the one factor that makes them seem to defy gravity, creating that beautiful illusion of growing from the top down, and not the other way around. The vertical support system also reduces the possibility of fungal diseases on the plants, due to the presence of improved air circulation or proper ventilation around the plants. Just think about a hanging garden, defying gravity without any obscurity of fungal diseases, that is true beauty which this tip easily offers to you.

Make Use of a pH Testing Kit

pH testing kits determine the acidity or alkalinity of the soil which plants grow in the hydroponic system; their use is essential to the nutrient availability of plants. An optimum range for plant soil is 5.5 -6. Which is neither basic nor acidic, but neutral enough for the plant to grow. For plants not to have nutrient deficiencies, the use of a pH system is highly recommended.

Apply Compost Annually to Your Garden

Plants draw nutrients from soil, and this alone reduces the richness of the soil used in cultivating the crops because they deplete with time. One way to ensure that the soil regain these lush nutrients that it once offered your plants, is to allow it either fallow or add compost to it. These ensures the soil is rich enough in nutrients which the plants need.

Install Garden Netting

Nets are protective covers for young crops from insects, birds and also animals that are more than willing to graze or chew your hard work in their tummies. Animals like cats, sheep and even tiny insects can easily destroy your hard work if you do not prevent them from doing so. And, if you don't want to use a protective net cover. Here's another tip that might prevent any heart breaks should your plants be eaten, don't plant your garden. But, if you intend to, use a protective net cover.

Ensure Your Plants Have Access to Natural Lighting

Plants need natural light to grow because it helps with photosynthesis. If your garden does not have proper access to natural lighting, then they will be deficient, lacking the nutrients photosynthesis offers.

Take Extra Classes on Growing a Garden

It is necessary to add to the knowledge one has on a certain topic, no knowledge is lost, and these things you learn will come handy in the future. Take online classes, attend webinars, read books, find out the latest techniques in growing your own hydroponic garden, because this equips you to be at the forefront of planting gardens, and it also equips you with current trends in the business, and also what the future holds. All these forms of information are needed, if your garden will be the talk of the town.

Final Words

We've come a long way throughout the course of this book. Starting with a definition of hydroponics, we're covered a lot of information that will help you to get started on your own hydroponic garden. Before we close, let's go over a brief summary of what we covered and share some words on where to go from here.

Hydroponics has been around for literally ages, but it is only just starting to pick up some serious interest. These gardens can take a bit of work to set up and maintain but they offer a great way of growing crops. We focused here on those looking to get started with hydroponics, so we tailored our information towards the beginner. The lessons we covered, however, have everything the beginner needs to get started and begin the road to expert.

We have six primary setups to choose from when it comes to what kind of system we want to set up. We saw how to set up deep water, wicking and drip systems. These are the easiest systems for DIY setups and beginners but there are also aeroponics, ebb and flow and nutrient film technique systems. These systems are more complicated than is recommended for a beginner one, but I encourage you to research these more as you get more comfortable with hydroponics.

There are four key elements that we looked at as the operation cycle of the hydroponic garden. These are soiling, seeding, lighting and trimming. By understanding how each of these elements works, we are able to handle the growing cycle of our plants. There are many options available for soiling and several for lighting. Finding the combination that is right for you will take some research, but it should ultimately be decided on what plants you want to grow.

Speaking of plants, we have seen that there are a ton of plants that work really well in hydroponic gardens. Herbs grown in a hydroponic garden have 30% more aromatic oils than those grown in soil. Lettuce in particular absolutely adores growing hydroponically. Each plant has its own preferences when it comes to how much water it wants, the pH level it likes best and the temperature that it needs to grow. For this reason, we have to research our plants and make sure that we only grow those that are compatible together.

The importance of maintaining a clean garden cannot be stressed enough and so we spent time learning how we care for our gardens. To do this, look at how often each step of maintenance needs to be performed and plan ahead so that you don't forget. It's super important that we take care of our plants because we don't want them in dirty environments, nor do we want them to be overly stressed. A dirty environment and a stressed plant are a recipe for infestation and infection.

Infection is a risk with all gardens and so our number one tool in preventing harmful pathogens from attacking our plants is to make sure that our plants are nice and strong. We clean our gardens, we provide them with nutrients mixed to their liking, we give them the love and care they need and in doing this we keep them healthy and unstressed. While infection can still take hold in a healthy plant, it is far more likely to attack stressed plants.

Finally, we looked at mistakes that are common to beginning hydroponic gardeners. We also exploded those myths that surround hydroponics to dispel the lies and untruths surrounding our newfound hobby. Searching online for tips or mistakes will reveal many discussions with hydroponic gardeners that are written specifically to help beginners like you to have the easiest, most enjoyable time possible getting into this form of gardening.

If you're excited to get started, then I suggest you begin planning out your garden now. You will need to dedicate a space for it and pick which system is most appealing to you and your skill level. Write down the plants you are most interested in growing and begin gathering information about them; what environment do they like best? What temperature? How much light do they need? What pH level?

Once you know what plants you want to grow and what system you want, you can start to build a shopping list. Along with the hardware to set up the system itself, don't forget to get some pH testing kits and an EC meter. Also make sure you have cleaning material, as you know now how important it is to sanitize and sterilize your equipment. This is also a great time to build your maintenance schedule.

Once you have this information you can return to this guidebook and use it as a manual for walking through every step of the growing process. The information that we covered will take you from beginner and, along with the application of practice, turn you into a pro in no time. But most importantly, don't forget to have fun!

CPSIA information can be obtained
at www.ICGtesting.com
Printed in the USA
LVHW081333251020
669606LV00014B/816